Living with an Oil Sensitivity

Avoiding Industrial Seed Oils

By Celina Thomas

Disclaimer

I am not a doctor. This book is not intended as a substitute for the medical advice of physicians. The reader is advised to regularly consult a physician in matters relating to his/her health and particularly with respect to any symptoms that may require diagnosis or medical attention.

Table of Contents

Introduction

This is the book I wish my mother had found back in the 1990s when she first realized that some of my intestinal issues were caused by oils. We did not understand how to avoid oils, nor did we comprehend just how hard they were on my health. In my ignorance, I ate them for many more years, and it is probable that many of my subsequent health problems could have been avoided if I'd only known then what I now know. My hope is that by sharing what I've learned in this book, I can help others access information that can make a difference in their health, allowing them to live happier, fuller lives.

This book is not meant to convince anyone to start an oil free diet. It is for people who have already decided that industrial oils might be a problem for them. In this book, I show what an oil sensitivity can look like and then talk about where industrial food oils are found and how one can go about avoiding them. It's a practical how to guide.

If you need to be convinced that industrial oils are not a health food or that they can be a problem for the human body, please check out some of the books in my bibliography or do some research into how oils are made and the science of how they affect the human body. It can seem incomprehensible that a substance that is so ubiquitous in modern life can cause problems, and ludicrous that if this is the case that no one is aware of it. But I assure you scientists have been aware of the dangers of industrial seed oils since they were first manufactured. People who work with these oils are aware of their dangers and many people just like me are aware that they can make people sick. It took me a long time to decide to give up oils entirely and to realize that they were bad for me, and really, the only thing that completely convinced me was seeing my transformation from sick to healthy when I stopped eating them.

I include a section about what my oil allergy/intolerance looks like and a section about symptoms because it can be helpful and encouraging to see what other people are dealing with and confirm that you are on the right path, especially for those who are unsure if their difficulties stem from an oil sensitivity or something else.

There are many reasons for avoiding oils. Most of them are health related. People who are afflicted with cancer might want to avoid vegetable oils due to the known cancer-causing and accelerating effects of such oils. Allergies or sensitivities make it essential to avoid certain ingredients, be they GMOs, corn, soy or what have you. There has been some evidence that oils affect fetus growth. Pregnant women may choose not to eat them as a precautionary measure. People with kidney problems are often told to avoid industrial seed oils. Many diets advise avoiding these oils. Some people have problems with one or another of the industrial oils but not all of them. I have read about people who can't eat olive oil or canola oil, a.k.a. rapeseed oil. The thing is, these oils are ubiquitous in our modern world and they are often are found in unexpected places or not listed on labels.

Since I recognized my sensitivity in 2010, I have learned much via trial and error about this frustrating state of affairs. Avoiding oils can be difficult and time consuming. Thankfully, now that I am further along the learning curve, I have reached a place that I manage to stay away from oils for longer and longer periods of time. I'm hoping that this book will allow others to reach that safe plateau sooner rather than later.

I would like to point out that I live in the United States and my information is skewed toward what I know about personally. Labeling laws differ widely between countries and even states. Still, food manufacturers and retailers are global entities and my correspondence with people around the world confirms my suspicion that manufactured food and actual food production methods are similar worldwide. It is important for anyone avoiding industrial seed oils to research all foods that are consumed and products that are used, because manufacturers change their common practices regularly and laws change swiftly.

According to the Asthma and Allergy Foundation of America (AAFA), there are immunoglobulin E (IgE) mediated reactions and non-IgE mediated immune reactions. Both are reactions caused by the immune system and can cause unpleasant symptoms. However, IgE is responsible for what we typically think of as classic allergy with hives and anaphylaxis.

As far as I can tell, the IgE is the most well studied of the immunoglobulins, but there are other *equally strong* antibodies that can affect the immune system, causing reactions that science is only starting to understand. The consensus in the medical literature seems to be that an intolerance involves difficulty digesting a food, an allergy involves an IgE reaction to a food, and a sensitivity can involve any immune reaction, including those not IgE-mediated, and intolerances. In this book, I use the term 'sensitivity' because it is often used as an umbrella term for both allergies and intolerances.

Over the years since I posted about my oil sensitivity in 2013 (at https://silverpenblog.wordpress.com), over 40,000 people have searched for and found my post. Numerous people have commented, and I have corresponded with many of them over the years. It has convinced me that I am not alone in my difficulties with oils and my struggles to avoid them. I am always learning new things, and I try to share that new information on my blog.

Much of the information in this book is on my blog in a less organized fashion. Thus, it is available for free to people who cannot afford to buy this book. This book was a labor of love. To keep the cost down, I did not hire a professional editor, so there might be some grammar and punctuation mistakes. If you have bought this book, know that you are supporting my writing and blogging efforts. Thank you!

Disclaimer

I am not a doctor. This book is not intended as a substitute for the medical advice of physicians. The reader is advised to regularly consult a physician in matters relating to his/her health and particularly with respect to any symptoms that may require diagnosis or medical attention.

Chapter One: The Discovery

I discovered my sensitivity to oils twice: once as a child and again as an adult. Hind sight is always twenty-twenty, so it's easy to see now that if I had realized how important it was to keep oils out of my diet that first time, I might have saved myself much misery and trouble later in life, but unfortunately, neither my mother, who detected the problem, nor I, were aware of the importance or the difficulties of avoidance and I had to discover my problem a second time with a new understanding of what it meant before that importance sank in.

My sensitivity may have been going on my entire life. As a baby I had issues with formula. Formula almost always contains industrial seed oils. My mother often told me about the goat lady whom she had to buy milk from since it was the only milk besides breast milk that I could keep down.

As a child, I had sinus infections regularly, along with cramps, gas and diarrhea. When I was around the age of ten, my mother ran out of Crisco one evening and used butter to make my favorite meal of hash browns and ham. She subsequently noticed that I did not have my habitual horrible smelly and acutely painful gas. She tried using Crisco again and the gas returned with a vengeance. Further experimentation showed that when she used butter, I seemed to be fine. Even though she was surprised by the effect, she removed Crisco and other industrial cooking oils from our home, cooking with butter instead. I was happy not to have such appalling gas anymore. This was the first 'discovery'. My mom did some research but there was absolutely nothing in the literature at the time about people having problems with oils or fats. Prominent in the literature, ironically, was the assurance that childhood digestive and allergic issues resolved once the child grew up. Having no idea of the prevalence of industrial seed oils in food products, we did not start reading labels and I continued to eat processed foods and restaurant foods with no consideration of how they were prepared or what was in them.

I did suffer from bouts of gas, but I guess I never thought it was serious enough to stop eating the foods that I thought I loved. I was even happy when my constant diarrhea later morphed into constipation, because I didn't need to run to the bathroom as often and I had no idea what healthy bowel movements looked like.

I also had learning difficulties. Although never diagnosed, I had all the symptoms of dyslexia. I had trouble learning to read and even though I could draw very well, handwriting was hard for me. I could not seem to remember which way letters and numbers were supposed to sit on the page.

My mother also noticed that I would forget things I had learned with scary thoroughness. I would learn things one day and have them down pat – only to find them completely gone a day or two later; I would not even remember that I had known them. For example, we discussed how to divide a cup of sugar in half for a recipe one week, and the next week making the same recipe I would have no recollection of the conversation. My mother found it odd. There seemed little rhyme or reason to my mental blips, and I was unaware that they were happening. This made memorization difficult if not impossible.

General cognitive tasks such as counting down from a hundred, remembering strings of numbers, or any other short-term memory functions were very hard for me, as well. School brought many of those difficulties into sharp relief. Although some teachers were kind to me, my general impression of school was one of utter indifference to my needs. There were some difficult parent teacher conferences and I was nearly held back a grade.

Even as a small child I suffered from what my mother and I called bouts of 'the end of the world'. An 'end of the world' bout was characterized by feelings of abject misery and uncertainty about everything in life. These bouts would come on suddenly and unexpectedly and there would usually be no concrete reason for the feelings: nothing bad had happened, there was no new stress, and no one had been mean or unfair. The bouts would end as suddenly as they came on. The only thing my mother could do was comfort me until the feelings had passed. I hid my feelings from friends and extended family because I thought the bouts meant I was crazy.

Eventually I graduated high school and moved to Seattle. Like most people that age, I got a low paying job and basically mistreated myself by staying up late, drinking, and eating poorly. I still had stomach issues and "end of the world" bouts and it became obvious to me that I was frailer than the people I spent time with. I was sensitive to stress and could not drink as much or stay up as late, but I pushed my limits as far as they would go.

In some ways, my health issues made me a bit of a character in my social circle. I had a white diet consisting of mostly carbs and refined sugars, which I now recognize is a sign of not being able to digest protein well. I was also known for falling asleep at parties, in moving cars, or even on my lunch hour at work on a cafe table because I needed more than twelve hours of sleep a day and I refused to miss out on fun.

During this time, I was eating a lot of processed foods which I now know contain processed oils. I also had blood sugar highs and lows, making me cranky, tired, lethargic and prone to sugar cravings. I got away with this behavior for several years, but eventually my health deteriorated. I became chronically nauseous. The nausea turned into full-fledged vomiting for a few weeks but returned to nausea eventually. I caught every little cold that came around. I had eye problems, sick rashes, acne, sinusitis, hay fever, back problems, wrist and foot pain, headaches, premenstrual syndrome (PMS), anxiety, and, eventually, I became depressed. Ultimately, I moved back home with my mother.

At home, I did a little better because I took better care of myself. But my mother was very worried: I had no energy and I seemed to be getting worse rather than better.

I decided I was tired of being sick and set out to improve my health. To that end, I read all kinds of books about health and I tried many things, including improving my diet, taking medication for depression, and exercise. Some of it helped a bit, but I was still unthinkingly consuming oils.

We finally started to become aware of what was causing my issues after I ate a bagel that caused some horrible intestinal gas. I thought it was a terrible thing that something like a bagel that generally does not have any oil in it would set off my sensitivity to Crisco and other industrial oils. I did not think too much about it, but my mother was on the scent.

Christmas 2010 I got worse. I had belly cramps, cold sweats and nausea, and then I started throwing up. I thought it was the flu or perhaps I had eaten some bad food. But it did not get better. The vomiting abated somewhat but the nausea continued. It was worse in the mornings, but if I did not eat, I felt weak and faint. If I did manage to eat a few soda crackers, it would be a few hours before the nausea subsided enough that I could eat real food. This went on and on. All through January and then into February. People wondered if I was pregnant. The tests came back negative. I did not consult a doctor because the same thing had happened before in Seattle. When I had gone to the doctor about the vomiting, he had scratched his head, run some expensive tests and given me anti-nausea pills to help me get back to work. He did not have a clue about what was wrong with me and I could not see what good it would do to consult another doctor except to waste a lot of money. I was sure it would pass.

My mother was not content to let me suffer. In the middle of February, she read the ingredient list on the box of Bagel Bites that I had bought to try to tempt my appetite. It was right there on the box: canola oil. I had not checked. She did not even have to suggest that I start checking labels. I knew that canola oil did not agree with me and being as sick as I was, I could not afford to be further weakening myself with things that my stomach took exception to. I stopped eating the bagel bites.

When I realized that all store-bought breads listed soybean oil I wondered if soybean oil was a kind vegetable oil. Just in case, I stopped eating store bought bread and started eating only bread I made at home. I kept reading labels and finding that oils were in everything I had been eating. Tortillas had shortening, crackers had soybean oil, hash browns and French fries had vegetable oil. The more oil-soaked food I removed the better I felt. Not just better: amazingly better. It was clear to me that I was on the right track.

I no longer needed a nap in the afternoon. I did not feel exhausted from waking up in the morning. It was as if I were a different person, a normal person, a person who could go for longer than two hours without eating, someone who could make it through a whole day without collapsing, and then get up the next day and do it again without being sick as a dog. It took a few months off the oils for the acne on my back and my face to clear up, but it did clear up.

The most amazing part was how much sharper my thoughts were. Memories were more easily accessible; not only could I find where I had put my keys down or what came next in a recipe, but things I had never been able to do with ease started being easy, such as spelling. My ability to learn increased exponentially. I even started teaching myself French and was doing quite well.

Then I made a mistake. I went out for breakfast. Within hours I felt tired, my guts began to cramp, a cold sweat broke out, and I wanted to sit down and cry. Soon I was exhausted and vomiting. It took two days for me to start feeling better. Subsequent exposures have taken longer to recover from. Every time I've been exposed, my "learning disability" returns full force, only to recede again when I stay away from the oils.

It turns out that my "end of the world" bouts were the first symptom of an exposure to oil. I had not been crazy as I'd worried; it was simply my body's initial reaction to what it perceived as a toxin.

I am grateful that my mother decided early on to support me by making sure all our shared meals were "Celina safe." She still ate oils in her work lunch, but the fact that she shared my diet made it easier for me, and safer. At that time, the only food in the house that we knew contained oils were the potato chips my mother had in her lunch each day.

Eventually we realized that, although we had gotten most of the oils out of my diet, we were not sure we had gotten all of them. We decided to try an elimination diet. It was a fancy one, banning all the top allergens. That lasted all of two weeks, but in that time, we did discover that olive oil was a problem for me, although a much subtler one than other oils. Also, my mother discovered that she did not really miss her lunch time potato chips. After that, she went completely oil free.

Six months later I started noticing a difference in her. It was subtle at first but grew more pronounced. Her memory improved. Remembering things started being easier: what she had had for dinner the night before, a show we had watched. The benign tremor that had plagued her started to abate; she could now hold out her hand and it would not shake. Her balance improved enough that getting in and out of the car was less of a chore. The arthritis in her hands got enough better that she could knit again.

She has also experienced a huge improvement in her skin. Her dry skin has improved considerably.

In *Deep Nutrition* (Shanahan 2017) Catherine Shanahan writes that industrial seed oils lead to people having problems with sun exposure. My mother and I are both fair skinned, and it used to be that we burned almost instantly; now we can spend time in the sun without sunscreen.

Gluten sensitivities seem to be the closest in symptoms to what I experience when I eat oils. Interestingly, researchers of Celiac disease are finding that only a minority of people with an intolerance to gluten show intestinal symptoms. Most people intolerant to gluten show brain inflammation with no intestinal issues. I suspect oil sensitivities are similar in nature. It's possible that there are more people like my mother out there who have issues with processed oils, but only show the effects in their brains (and skin) rather than their guts.

After my incredible recovery, I spent a lot of time reading whatever I could find about oils and health. There was very little about allergies, and most of the literature claimed that seed oils are less of a problem than animal fats for people with allergies. I have been unable to find any evidence proving that. The theory seems to be based on the assumption that the body's immune system reacts to the proteins in foods and, because oils have no proteins, they 'should' not cause allergic reactions. This protein theory of allergic reaction is well entrenched, even though many of the studies coming out of over the past few years have not supported it.

Despite the lack of data about oil sensitivity, I did find out lots about the manufacturing and distribution of modern industrial seed oils. It was not reassuring. Modern oils are produced using complex processes that often involve toxic chemicals and they are usually not very clean or well taken care of during processing or shipping.

I also learned that industrially processed oils are a recent invention and are not the same as traditional fats. They look completely different at a molecular level, and scientists are finding out that they work differently in the body too. The long-term effects caused by industrial seed oils are only just beginning to be understood. This book does not cover the science behind what industrial oils do or why they are bad for people because not only would that would be a much longer book, but other people have already written about it. After much reading, I concluded that seed oils are not a health food and made a great effort to avoid them. I include a bibliography for anyone who is interested in reading further.

Chapter Two: How I Used to Eat Versus How I Eat Now

I include this chapter because I felt it was important that I be honest about the changes that I made in my diet in order to avoid oils. I do not believe that everyone must change their diet the way that I did, but I do believe some lifestyle change is impossible to avoid. Change does not have to be onerous; however, because industrial seed oils are so integral to the modern lifestyle it would be unrealistic to expect to keep a diet otherwise unchanged while removing them.

I choose to cook all of my own meals, except when trusted family or friends cook for me. I have contemplated what I would have chosen to do if I had lived alone or had to work outside the home and have realized that my choices would have been much different.

When I first discovered my food sensitivity to oils, both my mother and I were picky eaters, mostly because we were sick a lot. I tried to change our diets as little as possible so that we would continue to eat by making – oil free -- as many of the same foods that we had been eating ready-made or outside the home. The foods we liked were things that required a lot of time and effort to cook, such as lasagna. Because I was not working full-time, I spent more time planning and cooking than most people might be willing to do.

We did decide not to eat out as much. It was not terribly burdensome, as my mother found it as stressful as I did to make sure I ate oil free at local restaurants. We found it easier to eat at home, and so we did.

The actual content of our diet has shifted as well but that is not entirely because of the oil restriction.

I worried for a while that I was restricting my mother's diet and that she would be unhappy. However, as her health has improved on the oil-free diet I have stopped worrying. She tells me that she does not miss oils and in fact she feels more centered without them.

After eating oil free for several years and feeling better because of it, my diet has broadened. I am more willing try new foods and recipes. I am also less willing to cook large complicated recipes and do the subsequent piles of dishes. Now we eat mostly simple meals that require less preparation and attention, which is why I know that it is possible to cook less and eat all homemade food. This style of simple cooking is what I would probably have ended up with if I had been working when I had first discovered my sensitivity.

I would have also relied more heavily on the few prepared foods that do not contain oil, even though sometimes they may be hard to find. There are also many methods of food preparation that most people would not consider 'cooking' such as making soups, salads and sandwiches. Even homemade, these foods require very little effort to prepare. Many "snack" foods are also healthy and oil free. They too would be things that I would have used if I hadn't had so much free time to cook at the beginning. It is possible to avoid oils and not to spend your whole life in the kitchen preparing homemade foods. However, it is not possible to avoid thinking about food or knowing anything about how foods are prepared. Because of this, I would think that the transition to an oil free diet will always feel like a major change even if there are few changes to the actual substances that are consumed.

Chapter Three: Possible Reasons for an Oil Sensitivity and Why an Oil Elimination Diet Can Help

Over the years of writing my blog, I have heard from many people who are suffering from the effects of eating oils and/or fats that disagree with them and I have come to the reluctant conclusion that we are not all suffering from the same issues. Yes, oils and/or fats are a problem for us all, but the *reason* that they are an issue seems to vary quite a lot. Some of us are having primarily digestive issues, while others are suffering from anaphylactic symptoms, brain fog, mood changes, skin problems, and/or multiple food sensitivities to a huge range of foods in addition to oils. I've thought a lot about what might be causing such a wide spectrum of problems. Here are some of the reasons that I think oils and fats can be problematic.

For some people, it may be a digestive issue. Digesting fats can be difficult. There are many steps to the process and any number of things can get in the way. Then again, sometimes digestive problems can be caused by various issues in the body. Beyond the intestines, there are several organs that are involved in digestion. The pancreas, the thyroid, the gallbladder and the liver are all involved, and there are any number of reasons that they might not be working as well as they should.

Even blood sugar levels can affect digestion. Sugars can dissolve the helpful labels that your body places on fat molecules to tell other organs how to process them. Without labels or with distorted labels, the fats are incorrectly handled by the body or not handled at all, leading to dysfunction. (Shanahan 2017)

Another digestive issue is called leaky gut, where undigested particles of food move into the bloodstream or other areas foods don't belong and cause inflammation.

This can lead to food sensitivities and worse. Sometimes there are things that can be done to support the digestion in its efforts and close these holes so that support is needed only temporarily.

For other people, it may be one or more chemical sensitivities. Fats are great at delivering various substances to the body. Sometimes those are helpful substances (think vitamin D) and sometimes they are damaging to the body (think pesticides) and depending on how your body reacts to chemicals, large enough amounts can cause problems. Vegetable oils and their derivatives are loaded with chemicals. Vegetable oils are produced using chemicals such as hexanes, which can be particularly vicious. If this is a problem, usually other chemical exposures will be making a person sick as well.

Another possible source of trouble is distorted fat molecules. Fats are delicate structures and they interact with our body chemistry in intricate ways. Industrial processing methods can distort fats and cause problems. Processes that can cause issues include intense heat, light, hydrogenation, chemicals, etc. The more processed fats are, the more likely they are to be problematic for people—another reason that removing vegetable oils from the diet is helpful.

Not all fats are the same. Monounsaturated, polyunsaturated, saturated are broad categories that most people are aware exist. But within each category are a dozen or more different types of fat. The chemical profiles of different types of fats are staggering in their complexity. Naturally, each person reacts differently to these variations.

People can also be allergic to oils. I have read in several places on the web statements by doctors and scientists that it is impossible for the body to be allergic to fat because fats have no protein or very little. I am not sure how they arrived at the conclusion that it is impossible, but in the messy world we live in it does seem to be possible to be allergic to oils. I know of at least two people who have anaphylactic reactions to oils, both aerosolized and consumed.

Industrially processed oils are also made in large quantities and transferred in large containers that have transferred other things. They are not as clean and pure as portrayed in advertisements. This means that if a person has an allergic reaction it may be possible that the reaction is to a contaminant that the oil came in contact with during processing or shipping.

More recently I have read that many edible vegetable oils have heavy metals in them. Heavy metals such as mercury, aluminum, nickel, cadmium, arsenic, iron, and lead can all cause significant problems for healthy people in high amounts, but if a person is sick or compromised in some way or already dealing with heavy metal toxicity, adding more to their diet would be very bad.

I am sure I've missed other pathways by which oils can cause problems. If a person suffers when consuming oils, they will do better when oils are removed from their diet. For some, it is enough to banish one type of oil; for others, stringent avoidance of even the smallest speck of any type of oil is the only way to be symptom free.

My mom, for instance, does not have the symptoms that I do when she eats oils, but she thrives on an oil-free diet, possibly because she has other chemical sensitivities. Despite the different origins of our discomfort, the same treatment (the oil-free diet) is helpful for both of us.

If oils are a problem, I believe that there is a considerable benefit to reducing oils in the diet. However, even a tiny amount of oil a day might really mess up a person's health, although the effects can be masked by the normal ebb and flow of moods and life. Moods go up and down, our ability to deal with stress is constantly fluctuating, and humans are incredibly adaptable. We become used to feeling 'off' or 'having a bad memory', and we compensate. When improvements to memory or moods are slow and steady, we often do not recognize the fact that we are doing 20% better than we were last week. We only see that we are still not doing well.

The insidious thing about oils is that *the mental effects are not recognizable to the person being affected by them*. I myself was oblivious to the very heavy tolls that oils were having on my memory and moods until I had removed oils completely for long enough to be doing very well. It was only when I became sick after being well and saw the fact that I couldn't mentally do the things that I had been perfectly capable of doing the day before that I realized that I really had been better off the oils.

I would still believe that the benefits I see in my own life were unique to me if it were not for the improvements I have witnessed in my mother's health after complete removal of the oils. She still has bad days and memory problems, but she is much better than she was when she was eating the oils. We have also witnessed a revival of her earlier symptoms after oil exposures.

If I had to do things all over again, knowing what I know now, I would do a proper oil free diet: an elimination diet that focused solely on avoiding oils. I now know many more places that oils can be found that I slowly eliminated over time. Unfortunately, I cannot go back in time. I can only offer my hard-earned knowledge to others who are currently thinking that they have a problem with oils.

Even my slap dash oil elimination diet was effective because it made it easier to pinpoint what foods were causing symptoms. The human diet is so broad that it is really difficult to tell exactly what food or environmental substance is causing a problem. That is why doctors like tests. A good test can pinpoint the culprit that is causing a set of symptoms. Unfortunately, there are few good tests for food sensitivities, and there are none that I know of for oil sensitivity.

The only way I know of to find out if a person has an oil sensitivity is to eliminate oils from the diet and observe the results–essentially an oil elimination diet. If oils are a problem, taking them out should make a person feel better. If oils are a problem, reintroducing them will cause symptoms to resume.

For a while I worried that we *needed* to eat vegetable oils: after all, they are vigorously promoted as 'heart healthy'. My research has convinced me that, on the contrary, these oils (other than olive oil and coconut oil) are all relatively new to the human diet. None of our great, great grandparents ever ate them. They are not essential for human health, so it is just fine not to consume them. By eliminating them from our diet, we are not depriving ourselves of a health food.

While it is true that refined oils do contain Omega 6's and Omega 3's, whole foods, including flax seed, salmon, cod, sardines, eggs, and grass-fed beef, provide sufficient Omega 3's and 6's to keep us healthy. There is no need to eat oils to get essential fatty acids.

People are often sensitive to more than one substance. I am oil sensitive but also sensitive to gluten. My mother is also gluten sensitive. We both saw an improvement with an oil free diet, even though we were still eating gluten, unaware of our sensitivity to it. If oils are a problem for a person, that person should see some improvement on an oil free diet, even if they have other sensitivities. There are lots of books covering sensitivities to gluten, corn and nuts, so I am not going to address those allergens here. Suffice it to say, I feel that if there is "some" improvement from an oil free diet, oils are probably part of the problem.

Depending on the severity of symptoms, resolution can happen sooner (within a week, for me) or later (six months, for my mother), but a fair trial will last a least a month or two with no exposures.

Elimination diets have another positive effect besides the direct benefits of resolving (or not resolving) symptoms. I have been on a few such diets over the years– some more effective than others. The act of *doing* something is amazingly restorative. After years of suffering helplessly at the hands of illness, the act of taking charge, of researching foods, deciding what to put in my mouth and observing how it affected me, was incredibly empowering. It did not hurt that I found some foods that cause me problems. I think that one of the reasons that people go on diets is because of the sense of control that dieting gives a person.

Many people recommend using a food journal to log symptoms and foods eaten. This is a great idea, and if you can bring yourself to conscientiously write information down, this could be invaluable for tracking exposures and helping to show how foods affect you. I am very bad at keeping a log and have never managed to keep track of the foods I eat or my symptoms regularly enough for a food journal to help me. I even tried doing it with my smart phone to no avail.

I keep mentioning symptoms. It is a sad fact that one person's sensitivity will look very different from that of the next person, and a sensitivity to one food can look exactly like a sensitivity to another, completely different food. Keep that in mind when reviewing the following list of possible symptoms. Also, remember that I do not know all the possible symptoms that could be associated.

Possible Symptoms of Oil Sensitivity

For me, acute symptoms can be delayed anywhere from a few hours to several days. It only takes a trace of the offending substance to cause a severe reaction. The less acute symptoms can last anywhere from a few weeks to a few months.

Other people have mentioned symptoms appearing almost immediately after breathing in oil laden air, contact with oils, oil-containing lotions, make-ups, and perfumes, which are often carried on oil. Reaction times for these folks are not delayed and they start having symptoms within fifteen minutes.

For people like my mother who are not experiencing any gut reactions, symptoms can be subtle and hard to pin down, often manifesting in emotions like depression or in long term problems like benign tremor, or arthritis. These symptoms are far from instantaneous. It can be quite difficult to figure out what is causing them.

Symptoms vary from person to person, in both severity and number.

The following list includes both symptoms I have experienced myself and those that others have reported to me.

Stomach issues:

Abdominal pain

Bloating

Constipation

Cramping, mild to severe

Diarrhea

Gas

Heartburn

Indigestion

Nausea

Poor and/or slow digestion

Vomiting

Allergy Type Symptoms:

Anaphylaxis

Aches

Breathing issues

Cough

Dry skin

Eczema

Fatigue, especially after eating

Fever

Headache

Heightened allergies

Hives

Itchy mouth, throat, skin

Joint pain

Low grade infections

Low immunity (i.e., extended healing times, chronic conditions, no defense against illness)

Migraine

Overall inflammation

Pain and itching

Rashes

Sensitivity to light, noise, and temperature changes

Swelling (in joints, tonsils, face, glands, etc.)

Mental and Emotional Symptoms

Anxiety

Cognitive issues

Crying jags

Depression

Difficulty making decisions and/or reasoning

Drugged feelings (not in any way pleasant)

Feelings of self-loathing

Irritability

Loss of energy and drive

Loss of proprioception (the sense of how our bodies are positioned) and balance

Memory loss

Mental fog

Mood changes

Obsessive thoughts

Panic attacks

Thoughts bouncing around

Other symptoms include:

Back pain

Benign tremor

Blood sugar issues

Blurred vision

Body odor (sulfuric)

Bruising easily

Caustic sweat

Cold sweats

Fungal infections

Hormonal issues

Inability to heal

Inability to relax muscles

Jaw clenching

Muscle spasms

Neck pain

PMS

Shin splints

Sleep issues

Sties

Teeth grinding

Tooth sensitivity

Trembling

Tremors

Vision problems (spots, floaters, flashes, and/or difficulty transitioning between light and dark)

Wrist problems

Yeast infections

How Long Does It Take to Get Better?

One of the most commonly asked questions on my blog is "how long will it take to recover from an oil exposure?" Almost all the people who write to me say it takes them a long time. For me if I have an oil exposure, there is an initial period of vomiting, gastric cramping and distress that will take three to five days to abate. After that I will be weak and still feel sick, often for several weeks. Even though after that I am up and moving, I often don't feel 100% better for several months. If I get a cold or sinus infection, I will often take even longer to get better. There are some suggestions for helping with recovery in Chapter 5 under "Dealing with Accidental Oil Ingestion."

Chapter Four: Eliminating Oils from the Diet

Many of the dietary gurus and people at the forefront of nutrition research warn against consumption of industrial seed oils. I have been disappointed when the same authors recommend recipes or supplements that contain the very oils they said to avoid. Although they are aware of the dangers inherent in consuming oils, they are not aware of how completely these oils have infiltrated our food. The effects for most people occur way too far down the road to easily be associated with the cause, and oils are hidden very successfully in many products that most people would never imagine would contain them.

In this chapter, I assume that that you are interested in doing an oil elimination diet and want to eliminate all oils from your diet.

Over the years I've heard a lot of people say, "I have a problem with 'X' oil, but the other oils seem to be okay." I thought that, too, and so I suffered for a lot longer than I would have if I had just taken all oils out of my diet and my environment to begin with. Now that I'm off oils, it a lot easier to spot an exposure and track down a potential source. As it was, I removed triggers in a haphazard fashion and spent a lot of time being sick. Often the symptoms were low grade enough to fly under the radar until things finally got bad enough that I noticed them. It was also aggravating to have to go over my life with a fine-toothed comb again and again, having no idea of where to look, as I tracked down the oils in my life.

Even small amounts of offending foods can trigger reactions. If the reaction is an allergy or sensitivity, the body will start to react to smaller and smaller amounts of the food over time and possibly start reacting to other foods as well. I have certainly found this to be true in my own life.

I have found it is easier to remove just one type of food than many types of foods from my diet. The standard elimination diet calls for removing all of the top seven or eight known allergens as well as sugar, caffeine, tomatoes, chocolate, and, well… basically anything that people like to eat. It is really hard, and certain people get cranky when deprived of everything they like all at once.

The good news is that, while eliminating oils is not easy, oils do not add flavor or texture to food, so there is less of a feeling of deprivation with an oil-free diet than, say, a gluten-free diet or a standard elimination diet. It is fairly easy to make my favorite foods at home without oil.

The bad news is that there are not a lot of vegetable oil-free foods and body products available, so eliminating oils requires reading a lot of labels, cooking from scratch and eating at home for the duration of your trial, as well as putting aside and not using many body care products, laundry products, and home cleaning products that contain oils for the duration of the trial. It also requires a certain amount of vigilance when shopping that can be tiring.

When the trial period is finished, most elimination diets call for reintroducing foods one by one, spacing reintroductions by at least a week (longer if there is a bad reaction). On the few elimination diets that I have done, determining if illness was caused by a food or not was the most difficult part of a diet. Sadly, I learned no tricks to make that easier. As a lot of the effects of oils are cumulative, I think it would be very hard to determine if an oil is totally safe. As oils are not necessary to the human diet, I have refrained from intentionally reintroducing a lot of oils and oil products back into my life.

If you just want to remove large sources of oils, I do mention the amount of oil in each of the foods in the following pages which should allow you to decide if a food or product is worth avoiding.

A Note About Processed Foods

Processed foods are really a trick. I read labels religiously when I first discovered my sensitivity. Still, I kept getting sick. What I did not realize was that a lot of what I thought of as whole food was in fact processed food. Processed is a term that refers to altering or preparing a food for consumption. A can of tomatoes is indeed an ingredient for homemade food but originally, the contents were whole tomatoes that had to be peeled, chopped, cooked down and put into a can. Each step along the way can introduce new elements that we would never think would be in 'tomatoes'.

Even plain meat, vegetables and grains have been prepared in some way to make them look good on store shelves by being wrapped in plastic, covered in wax, or de-hulled. What I finally realized is that the food one buys will always be processed. The trick is not to avoid processed food, but to learn exactly what processing is likely to happen, and make sure that one can double check that there is no oil likely to be in that processing. That is much easier to do with minimally processed foods with few ingredients. A can of tomatoes is less processed than a can of spaghetti sauce, for example.

Surprisingly, oils are not always listed on the ingredient label when present in a food. It is important to check on the rest of the label for notes about processing equipment such as, "This was made on equipment that also came in contact with soy oil." Still, there are times when oils are not on the label at all or are disguised. I've run into more than one food that seems safe but in fact makes me sick. With time I have become better at predicting if a food will be safe for me but ultimately trial and error is always the name of the game.

Foods that Generally Do Not Contain Oils

The simplest way I've found to minimize exposure to oils is to start with whole, single ingredients, and then combine and cook them myself. Reading labels is a must. (See the section on label reading for things to watch for).

Meat– Simple, uncooked cuts straight from the butcher are best, with no added ingredients. Meat with broth added typically has dried onions and garlic in it but not listed; dried garlic and onions are usually contaminated with oils. Usually, oils are not used during cutting, but I checked that my butcher cleans the grinder between making sausage and grinding meat because sometimes sausage has oil laced flavorings. Most bacon is okay. Some sausage can be oil free, but I have found that sausage can contain orange juice and/or 'natural flavors' so I read labels carefully.

Fish– Fresh or frozen generally does not contain oils. Make sure that there are no additions such as broth. Some canned is fine when it is packed in water. I make sure to check the label.

Eggs– Fresh, whole eggs are oil free.

Tofu– Usually does not have oils added. I check the label.

Vegetables– Fresh, raw vegetables, preferably without plastic wrap. Frozen vegetables should list nothing besides the vegetable(s) on the ingredient list on the label. I tend to avoid canned vegetables because I do not know how they have been processed, but if the label does not list oils, I will occasionally eat them.

Fruit– Fresh, raw fruit. I will buy frozen fruit which lists only the fruit and perhaps sugar as ingredients; added sauces or other compound ingredients can have oils. I do not generally like canned fruits but if the label lists only fruit I would think they are safe.

Grains– I buy single ingredients such as flour, cornmeal, or rice. I make my own bread, cookies, pancakes, etc., from scratch.

Milk and some cheese– Pasteurized milk is fine for me, but I avoid homogenized milk. The homogenization process distorts the fats and these distorted fat molecules can provoke sensitivities even in people without an oil sensitivity. I check the label to make sure that nothing is added. Vitamin D is carried in a vegetable oil base. Also look out for oil derivatives such as mono and di-glycerides and polysorbate 80. Many dairy products such as yogurt, cottage cheese, sour cream, shredded cheese, and even cream can contain oil by-products such as polysorbate 80, so I read labels carefully. Longer lasting cheeses such as parmesan, cheddar, and mozzarella should be safe, but I avoid cheese products such as cheese in a can and processed 'cheese' like Velveeta, or cheese slices, as these often have oils or oil derivatives. Powdered milk is a product that may distort milk proteins, so I avoid them.

Ice cream– Some plain vanilla ice cream does not contain oil (e.g., Häagen-Dazs is safe as of this writing). Also some chocolate ice creams are fine. I double check flavored ice cream ingredients because some of the flavoring ingredients may be contaminated, even though no oil is listed. Citrus flavors are particularly bad about that.

Beans– Dry beans are safest but there are some vegetarian canned beans which do not contain oils. I read the label to make sure.

Nuts and seeds– Raw nuts and seeds are safe. Dry roasted might be safe; however, the salt might contain iodine which may be derived from palm oil. Most of the time I buy raw, then roast and salt my own.

Salt– I buy unrefined sea salt or pink Himalayan salt without added iodine, as iodine can be derived from palm oil. Later in the book I list some alternate sources of iodine.

Coconut milk– Many brands do not contain added oil. I double check the label.

Coffee– Coffee can be processed on equipment that is used for processing other foods. I buy Equal Exchange (I've called the company and asked about contamination; the equipment is used solely for EE coffee). I avoid anything with flavorings. Also, I grind and brew our coffee at home because the machines at stores and coffee houses are often contaminated with oils.

Tea– Plain black, green, white, and herbal teas can be safe. I avoid those that list soy lecithin or flavorings. 'Oil of Bergamot' is an oil, so I do not drink Earl Gray. Harder to check on but sometimes listed on the packaging is when tea is processed on equipment that has been processing other foods. Often, I just make herbal teas at home from plants I have grown because of this.

Kool-Aid– Can be safe but I look out for packets that list 'flavoring'.

Foods that Often Contain Oils

When I showed a list of what I needed to avoid to my dad, he looked at it, handed it back and said, "That's depressing! You basically can't eat anything."

His reaction surprised me because I do not think of it that way. Ingredients are called ingredients because they are building blocks of meals. Now that I cook everything for myself, I see lots of possibilities in whole, unprocessed foods for delicious creations. Sure, it is not as convenient as ready-made food, but I can make a huge variety of satisfying dishes from simple ingredients. Because I know I can cook (almost) any food that I might want from scratch, I do not feel deprived.

Still, this list of "can't haves" is a lot larger than the list of "can haves", so it can seem very overwhelming. Keep in mind that nearly everything offered in ready-made form at the store can be made oil-free at home, and that oil-free substitutes are available for things like iodized salt.

These are some of the foods in which processed oils can often be found.

Chocolate– A food group all by itself! Most eating chocolate contains soy lecithin or other vegetable oils. Even most baking chocolates are contaminated. While soy lecithin is an oil derivative and is not as destructive to my system as straight vegetable oils, it does cause me digestive issues. However, there are chocolates that do not contain oils. Any that contain only cacao butter, chocolate liquor, sugar and/or cocoa powder are safe! Cocoa powders are also free of oils at this writing. The higher the percentage of chocolate in a bar, the less likely it is to contain soy lecithin. I look for "Enjoy Life" and "Equal Exchange" chocolate and "Lindt" at 85% cocoa. Many flavored chocolates contain vegetable oils even if it is not listed as such, think of mint flavoring or raspberry. I read the label every time I buy.

Store bought broth– I've eaten store bought broth with no problem when it lists only broth; however, when used as an ingredient, broth generally contains powdered garlic and onions for flavor, these spices are often contaminated with oils and are not listed when broth is shown as an ingredient.

Pasta– I have never had an issue with eating dry pasta if it is not stuffed (e.g., ravioli); even the gluten free varieties have not bothered me. However, I have been told by people who have anaphylaxis that they always react to pasta, so it is possible that in the making of pasta machines are oiled and that oil comes in contact with the pasta.

Iodized Salt– Apparently iodine is often derived from palm oil. So, although I haven't noticed a problem with iodized salt, I do not like to take chances. I use unrefined sea salt. The Himalayan pink is particularly tasty. I haven't had any trouble with the lack of iodine, but I do eat seafood regularly. If lack of iodine is a problem, kelp is a natural source of it, which supplies several other minerals as well.

Alcohol– In many countries, including the U.S., there are no laws about contaminants. I have gotten sick because of this. The Europeans have more stringent laws. German beer and French wine are strictly controlled and probably safe. Remember that 'flavoring' is almost always associated with industrially produced oils, so I avoid any 'flavored' alcohol such as Crème de Menthe. Also, I recently read that during the making of certain wines, polysorbate 80 is used to keep foam down during brewing.

Juice and soda– I avoid these like the plague, especially citrus flavors. Manufacturers can add oils extracted from the skins of fruits without listing it on the label. They can also omit to mention chemical agents that have come in contact with the liquid.

Some 10% of citrus sodas in North America contain BVO (Brominated Vegetable

Oil). One of these sodas is Mountain Dew.

Soymilk, rice milk, and almond milk– Nearly all commercially available milk alternatives contain added oils (coconut milk is the exception here, probably because it is already full of coconut fat). It is very easy to make soy, rice or almond milk oil free at home with a good blender and a strainer. It also tastes better.

Frozen dinners, fish sticks, chicken nuggets, frozen French fries, etc.– I have found that 99% of these contain oil or oil by-products. The ingredients lists are very long on these.

Prepared meats– Many prepared meats are cooked in oil. Ham, rotisserie chickens, lunch meats, some bacon, sausages, potted and canned meats. Even in restaurants, meats are routinely marinated and/or seared in vegetable oils. I have to beware in the deli, as cross-contamination is a huge issue there. Also, delis, like bakeries, do not have to mention the oil that meats have been cooked in on the label.

Potato chips– Even if chips are baked, not fried, they contain oil.

Breads, cakes, pies, pastries, donuts, crackers and cookies– In bakeries, vegetable oil is usually chosen over butter or lard, probably because it is less expensive. Frosting is especially rich in oil or hydrogenated fats. I make my own from scratch at home with butter. Bread may not list oil in the ingredients, but the pan it was cooked in could have been greased with any kind of processed oils. By law, that oil does not have to be listed. Also, bulk yeast is often coated in an oil derivative called sorbitan monostearate. If yeast is listed on the ingredient list, it is most likely bulk yeast and does not have to list the sorbitan monostearate in its ingredients. I discuss bread in more depth in Chapter 5 Special Considerations.

Nuts (roasted)– Nuts are generally roasted in oil. It is possible to find dry roasted nuts and they seem to be fine for me, although there have been some notable exceptions. I find it super easy to soak raw nuts and roast them at home in the oven.

Pasta sauces– Both dry mixes and ready-made sauces in jars usually contain oils. (This is another item that is super easy to make at home, and very tasty).

Canned fish packed in oil–Oil is listed right there on the label.

Canned beans– Most are cooked in oils. I look for vegetarian, which are sometimes oil free.

Canned soup– Almost all canned soup contains oil.

Yoghurt– Yoghurt should be a pure food, but most brands have mono- and di-glycerides added.

Cottage cheese, sour cream– These used to be relatively safe products, but these days I have been finding more and more ingredients listed on the label such as mono- and di-glycerides.

Cream– There are a few brands which do not have mono- and di-glycerides and/or polysorbate-80. I check the label.

Mayonnaise– Mayonnaise is made with oil. I have not found a brand without. This is one thing that I have been unable to make at home with "safe" fats despite numerous recipes.

Salad dressings– Always made with oil by manufacturers. I easily make my own at home with butter or lard. It's a little strange looking, but very tasty.

Condiments– I am extra careful with these. They tend to have long lists of ingredients and it is easy to miss the oil or oil by-product hiding three-quarters of the way through.

Any kind of fake food such as egg substitutes or soy "cheese"– These will usually have oils.

Cooking spray– Any kind of cooking spray contains processed oils. These are particularly troublesome for people sensitive to aerosolized oils.

Bulk Yeast– If yeast is left out in oxygen it goes bad, thus manufacturers cover yeast that will be touching air with the oil derivative sorbitan monostearate to protect it. All bulk yeast is sold this way. If the yeast is sold in small air sealed packets, the sorbitan monostearate may not be added. I check the ingredient label.

Plastic– Oils are impossible to remove from plastic, so I avoid secondhand plastic equipment. Read more about this in the Cross- Contamination section.

Dried or powdered onions and garlic– (a.k.a. garlic or onion salt) I have been sick from these ingredients but because the amounts of oil used in the drying process is so small my reaction was hard to spot and it took me years to figure out what was going on. Other people have told me that their reactions are more severe.

Peanut Butter– Most common peanut butter brands list vegetable oil or palm oil on the label. However, when peanut butter is used as an ingredient, oil will not be listed on the label even if it is in the food. There are a few brands of peanut butter that have not had vegetable oil added, such as Adams Old-Fashioned. They generally have no added sugar either, so that's a bonus.

Reading Labels

It may sound like overkill, but I try to read the label on everything I buy every time

I buy it, both when I put it in my shopping basket and before I eat it. I do not know how many times I have mistakenly bought items that contain oils because I was tired or distracted. I like to have that extra check before I put stuff in my mouth, especially since products are liable to change. One bottle of tomato paste from the same company will not list oils, the next one will. I have been sick many times because of this ever-morphing landscape.

Label reading trick: the ingredient list is only one place to check. The rest of the label can contain valuable information. I look out for sentences like "This product processed on the same equipment used to process soy oil" in tiny print somewhere on the label. It will not be on the ingredient list.

If you do not want to try to memorize this list or copy it out, there is a shortened alphabetized list in the appendix.

Animal Fats and Hydrogenation

I seem to have no problem eating animal fats as long as they are not hydrogenated. However, several people have written to me saying that they cannot eat one type of animal fat or another, i.e., they can tolerate chicken fat, but pork fat seems to bother them. There are a few reasons this may be the case. People can be allergic to certain animal meats such as in alpha-gal syndrome, so I would assume the fat of the same animals would cause reactions as well. In addition, every animal fat has a different profile of saturated to unsaturated which, again, could cause issues. I've read about people who can't eat conventionally raised animals who can eat organic. Also, when meat is processed there are certain sanitizers and chemicals used in abattoirs, so it may not be the meat or fat per se that is causing issues. If meat fats seem to bother you it is probably best to avoid them. I do know that lard and other animal fats are often hydrogenated or partially hydrogenated to keep them shelf stable. It will generally be stated on the label. I have a terrible reaction to fats that have been hydrogenated.

Because of the hype about trans fats and their health consequences food manufacturers have turned to other methods of changing liquid vegetable oils into solids. One of those methods in called interesterification. Unfortunately, the fact that a fat has been interesterified does not currently have to be stated on labels in the US, Canada or in the United kingdoms but interesterified fats should be avoidable because they will be listed as the original vegetable oil or called something general such as "shortening".

Easy to spot oils

These say "oil" or "fat" in the name, making them easier to spot. Many kinds of solid fats are listed as "shortening" this is a catch all term that can encompass anything from Crisco to hydrogenated or interesterified fats. Because of the uproar over trans-fats, most countries' laws insist that labels must indicate if fats have been hydrogenated; not so for interesterified fats. Also, margarine or other butter-like spreads all contain oils of various types. I do not eat any fat that has been hydrogenated or partially hydrogenated or interesterified, as the fats have been altered, and are as a result unstable and potentially problematic.

Butter oil (not simply butter: this is butter that has been processed)

Canola oil, a.k.a. rapeseed oil

Cottonseed oil

Crisco

Grape seed oil

Hydrogenated oil, or partially hydrogenated

Light olive oil (always has been cut with canola or other vegetable oils)

Milk fat

Safflower oil

Sesame oil

Soybean oil

Sunflower oil

Vegetable oil

Nut oils, such as almond, walnut, pecan, and hazelnut

Flax oil

Avocado oil

Notice that nut oils, flax oil, and avocado oil are on the list. Even though they are considered healthy oils by many, Catherine Shanahan (Shanahan 2017) says many of these oils are very unstable and, due to the processes that are usually used to obtain them, the fats are distorted. They might have wonderful health benefits when fresh but from a store, these oils are little better than cheap industrial seed oils.

Coconut Oil & Palm Oil

In the case of palm oil and coconut oil, I have been told that they are healthy for most people as they are medium chain fats. The only thing is, I have been grievously ill from eating them. Your mileage may vary.

Extra Virgin Olive Oil

I have been told by many people that they can eat olive oil but none of the other industrial oils, but I have also been told the reverse is true for other people, so I would probably suggest avoiding it on an elimination diet and only add it back in to the diet when there is a good chance that the symptoms would be easy to spot.

Olive oil is different from industrial oils in several important ways. For one thing, it is mostly monounsaturated oil, rather than polyunsaturated. The second thing is that olive oil can be extracted from olives without the chemicals and high heat that other oils need.

In *Extra Virginity: The Sublime and Scandalous World of Olive Oil.* (Mueller 2013) Tom Mueller talks about how most experts agree that olive oil is a healthy oil; however, much like nut oils, it is unstable. It lasts one year if kept away from light, heat and oxygen. Most of the time, oil on store shelves is much older than a year. Moreover, many of these oils are not bottled in the correct kind of dark glass. The bigger issue is that oil is not a regulated market and much of what is sold as 'extra virgin olive oil' may not be. Much of it is contaminated with cheaper oils or outright fake. Even if it is 100% olive oil, the processes used to make it are far removed from the processes used traditionally: even some small-scale producers have machines that look like they were made by Dr. Seuss. Because my "100% extra virgin oil" made me sick, I avoid olive oils.

Hidden Oils

One good place to look out for hidden ingredients is flowing/anti-caking agents, which are often put in sugars, salts, and spices to make them flow better. Onion and garlic powders and salts are an example of this. Sanitizers/disinfectants are often used on machinery or equipment. Thankfully most sanitizers do not contain oil. On packaging, oils can be added to the insides of packages especially with bread products that might stick. In any kind of preservation, canned or dried food products often add oils to prevent sticking. If a product is fortified, remember many of the vitamins themselves are made from or floated in oils. Vitamin D is a good example. Fermentation products can also add all kinds of hidden ingredients. Often, hidden ingredients are not oils, but it is important to make sure.

These are some of the ingredients that are listed in food items and cosmetics that are derived from oils and fats which I avoid.

Acetaldehyde– Derived from coal tar or crude oil.

Alpha-linolenic acid– Derived from vegetable oils, do not confuse with alpha lipoic acid or linolenic acid.

Anhydrous milk fat– A shelf stable fat made from butter or cream using heat, mechanical action and a centrifuge. Similar to butter oil.

Blue #1– Although this was originally derived from coal tar, most manufacturers now make it from a vegetable oil base.

Brominated Vegetable Oil (BVO)– Banned for use in food throughout Europe and Japan, BOV is vegetable oil bonded to the element bromine. Bromine is an endocrine disruptor and competes for the same receptor cells that the human body uses for iodine.

BOV is found in about 10 percent of citrus flavored sodas in North America, including Mountain Dew.

Calcium laurate– is a combination of lauric acid and calcium. Lauric acid is derived from fats and oils.

Cis-vaccenic acid– A monounsaturated fat generally derived from animal fats or plant oils.

Dodecanoic acid– a.k.a. lauric acid is a saturated fatty acid which occurs naturally in various plant and animal fats and oils.

Docosahexaenoic acid (DHA)– A chemical name for fat, it is often derived from vegetable oils.

Gamma-linolenic acid (GLA) a.k.a. gamolenic acid– Derived from vegetable oils.

Glyceryl stearate– This can be derived from several possible sources: palm kernel oil, soy oil, or vegetable oil among them. Usually found in soap and cosmetics.

Glycerol– A fatty acid derived from plants and animals.

Hypromellose– An emulsifier that might be derived from oils.

Hydrogen cyanide– Derived from coal tar or crude oil.

Lactic acid (synthetic)– Made from acetaldehyde and hydrogen cyanide that are derived from coal tar or crude oil.

Lauric acid– a.k.a. dodecanoic acid is a saturated fatty acid which occurs naturally in various plant and animal fats and oils.

Linoleic acid– Derived from vegetable oils.

Lecithin– Generally derived from the manufacture of corn or soy oil. Used as a supplement as well as being used in chocolate.

Magnesium stearate– A derivative of stearic acid, where they take two molecules of stearic acid and bind them to magnesium to make a salt. Derived from animal or vegetable oils.

Mono- and Di-glycerides– A short chain of fatty acids. Used as emulsifying agent. Although technically fats, mono- and di-glycerides are not included in total fat on the "Nutrition Breakdown" panels of packaged foods.

Milk fat– Highly processed fat derived from milk or cream. This makes me very sick.

Octadecanoic acid– Chemical fat name.

Oleic acid– This is an umbrella term for most fats inside of plants. From the Greek for 'olive.' Oleic acid is classified as a monounsaturated omega-9 fatty acid. Derived from animal fats and plant oils.

Palmitoleic acid– It is a monounsaturated fat that can be derived from animal fats or vegetable oils.

Palmitoleic ascorbate– a.k.a. vitamin C ester, is a fat-soluble form of vitamin C usually made with vegetable oils.

Petroleum jelly– A petroleum product derived from fossil fuels (a.k.a. oil).

Polyglycerol polyricinoleate (PGPR)– PGPR is an emulsifier made from castor oil or soybean oil and is commonly added to cheap chocolate.

Polypropylene glycol stearyl ethers– Produced from the reaction of propylene oxide with stearyl alcohol. Stearyl alcohols are derived from animal fats and oils. Usually found in soap and cosmetics.

Polysorbate 20 and polysorbate 80– Polysorbate 20 a.k.a. Tween 20, Scattics, and Alkest TW, is a polyoxyethylene derivative of sorbitan monolaurate and is used as a detergent, emulsifier and wetting agent. It is derived from fats. Usually found in soap and cosmetics. I have seen three different numbers after the label polysorbate, the '80' usually in cream. I assume that they are all made in a similar fashion. Also found in injections and vaccines.

Simethicone– "Wikipedia" says that it is an anti-foaming agent made of polydimethylsiloxane and hydrated silica gel. Silica comes from rocks. Polydimethylsiloxane belongs to a group of chemicals called silicones, and specifically a branch called silicone oils. Apparently, silicone oils are not absorbed by the human body and thus are considered safe for human consumption. Usually found in Gas X, and other anti-gas products.

Sodium stearate– This is a very old chemical used for centuries. It is produced as a major component of soap upon saponification of oils and fats. Saponification is the chemical change of fat into soap. Usually found in soap and deodorant. This is one of the few things on this list I still use, but only externally.

Soy lecithin– Generally, soy lecithin contains about 35% soybean oil and 16% phosphatidylcholine. It is a by-product of the soy oil making process and is found in many food products, especially chocolate.

Sorbitan monostearate– An oil derivative usually made from corn that is used on bulk yeast to protect it from oxygen.

Stearic acid– Derived from animal fats or vegetable oils.

Stearyl alcohols– Derived from animal fats or vegetable oils. Usually found in soap and cosmetics.

Triglycerides– Derived from animal fats or vegetable oils.

Vegetable stearin– Glycerol and stearic acid derived from animal and vegetable fats.

Vegetable glycerin– a.k.a. glycerol or glycerin, is typically made from soybean, coconut or palm oils.

Fish Oil

Fish oil is a very popular supplement right now in paleo and natural health circles. My grandmother had to take cod liver oil when she was a child. The Weston Price Foundation points to research that shows taking fish oil helps heal dental cavities. Also, it is commonly used to boost essential fatty acids (Omega 3's) and vitamin D.

I took a cod liver oil for a while, but I worried about how it was processed and stopped taking it. Only to start taking a different brand when I needed omega 3s for pregnancy, this time in a capsule. I took Vital Choice sockeye salmon oil in capsules with no bad effects until they changed the formulation of their pills. They added glycerin (an oil byproduct) and lemon oil to their pills, which did cause me very slight stomach symptoms over time. According to their website they use molecular distillation to purify their oils. Many manufacturers adulterate their fish oils with flavors or butter oil and add extra oil-based vitamins. These are usually stated on the front of the bottle and are easy enough to avoid, but manufacturers also seem to add many other things and only list them on the back in the ingredient list which I have forgotten to check. Things I have found include, d-alpha tocopherol, which is generally made from vegetable oils and rosemary extract which really upsets my digestion. It's important to be really careful

46

about buying fish oil and make sure to re-read every label before consuming.

I have switched to buying fermented cod liver oil because there is one company that sells it without any flavorings or additions. It is by Green Pasture and called Blue Ice Fermented cod liver oil. I have tried it and it seems to be okay for me. It does have a fishy taste and it also has a burn at the back of the throat which is unpleasant but goes away quickly with food. It does cause fishy burps after eating but they are not that bad.

My reading tells me that fermented cod liver oil is the traditional method of producing oil in a low temperature way. The bacterial process actually preserves the oil just like bacteria ferments cheese.

The molecular distillation process is harder to understand but from my reading on Wikipedia it sounds like they force oils into a small tube and use vacuum pressure and the subsequent heat it produces to encourage the particulates like mercury and other heavy metals to leave the oil in a continuous stream. Despite the mention of high heat, somehow this process does not damage the delicate fats. As I said earlier, I have not had any issues with my stomach after taking distilled fish oil when it is not adulterated. Unfortunately, I have been unable to find a variety of distilled fish oil that is not adulterated with some sort of vegetable oil derivative.

Because fish oil is an oil, I would not take it if I was trying out the oil free diet. However, given its history in promoting health, it would be one of the first oils I would try reintroducing at the conclusion of an oil free diet trial.

Other Fats

Fresh, unprocessed animal fats have had a bad rap, but new research is showing that they are vital for good health. I make sure to read labels and/or talk to the people who produce my fats to make sure they are not hydrogenated or treated with chemicals.

I have found the following fats to be safe for me to eat, but other people have told me that butter is a problem for them and even meat with extra fat gives some people difficulties. If you know that a fat gives you difficulties, you can avoid it.

Butter– Can be used in most every kind of cooking. Widely available.

Bacon Grease– Technically this is pig fat. It is something that most people cook out of bacon and throw away, but it is a wonderful fat for cooking. It can easily be saved in a jar and placed in the refrigerator for up to a month or in the freezer for up to a year before it is used (Mine never sticks around that long!) I use it in any savory dish that would commonly call for oil. Bacon grease is salty, but it is not difficult to adjust salt levels in a recipe to compensate.

Lard (a.k.a. Pig Fat)– Lard found at a grocery stores is generally hydrogenated and is *not* safe for me but lard which has not been hydrogenated or mixed with other fats or oils has never been a problem for me. I render mine at home. Rendering uses low heat to melt the fat out of the pig's flesh. It can be done using a crock pot or oven at home. I buy half a hog at a time and ask for the fat so that I can make lard. It makes stellar pie crust and lovely bread. I use it for greasing pans, sautéing, and just about anything that calls for oil or fat. I even use it melted in a warm salad dressing. It has a distinctive, pleasant odor and a mild taste. It keeps best in the freezer but keeps for up to a month in the fridge. I have found recently that I can buy lard at my co-op, but I have to be very careful because often producers add rosemary oil to the rendered fat to extend its shelf life.

Tallow (a.k.a. Beef Fat)– This is another fat that can be obtained through rendering. I have never been able to get more than a little of this fat at a time because butchers tend to trim off the excess fat, and I collect what cooks out of the meats I buy. Many people cook the fat out of hamburger only to throw it away. What a waste. Thicker and harder at room temperature than lard, this is a good fat for sautéing and adding flavor to any savory dish. I assume that buffalo and other ruminant fats are similar in texture. I find this fat to be particularly useful for any kind of homemade skin salve.

Schmaltz, (a.k.a. Chicken Fat)– I do not think you can buy this ready made in the U.S. I hoard the fat that comes off of cooked chickens and Cornish game hens and use it in many kinds of cooking. It is especially nice in bread. It has too much moisture for high temperature cooking but is fine for low heat sautéing and bread making. It also works well in savory pie crust.

Duck Fat– Duck fat is as close to lard as any other fat I have come across (goose fat is probably similar). It is low in moisture so there is less spitting when cooking at higher temperatures and it has a very mild flavor. One duck produces about a cup of fat as it roasts. I can buy several pounds of duck fat at the local co-op and keep it in my freezer.

Peanut Oil– I list this here because I have never suffered a problem from eating this oil. This may be because it is embarrassingly easy to get oil from peanuts. Grind them up and the oil separates. There's no need for expensive equipment, heat, toxic chemicals, or deodorizing agents. Unfortunately, many people have allergies to peanuts and peanut oil. Peanuts are a difficult food to digest and have lots of toxins both from the peanut plant and from the molds that can take up residence in them during transportation and storage. Because peanuts have a lot of arachidonic acid, most experts do not recommend this as a healthy oil. It is best not to fry with it or cook it at high temperatures as aerosolized peanut oil is linked to lung cancer. I don't think of it as an oil to be eating often, although in a pinch it could be used in hummus or as a substitute for other oils in salad dressing.

Cross Contamination

Cross contamination is when a substance that would ordinarily not be on a food or surface transfers onto it. Basically, any object can become contaminated with oils and then contaminate a person who is trying to avoid them. I have found it is best to not have vegetable oils or products containing vegetable oils in my home kitchen, even temporarily. Almost inevitably, if I eat in the same room as vegetable oil laden food, one way or another cross contamination occurs. I make sure all my food preparation surfaces and implements are oil free and make sure my foods do not share space with foods that contain oils. Researching celiac and other allergy cross contamination avoidance procedures really helped me to understand cross contamination in my kitchen and my life.

Deli Food

Many deli meats are cooked in vegetable oils. If it is in a sealed box with a label that does not list oil, I am 99% sure that there are no other ingredients in with the meat. However, if the meat is served at a deli there is a real chance that even if the ingredient list is clear, oil can easily transfer from the slicer or serving implements. It may seem obvious that meat and cheese the deli of a local supermarket is probably contaminated with oils even if the packaging does not list oil, but I made the mistake of eating food from there once. I even made the mistake of eating from a buffet and it made me sick even though the cook said that the foods I chose were not cooked with oil.

Kissing

Many of my early exposures were from my boyfriend. He would eat food that had vegetable oils in it, and we would kiss, sometimes several hours later, and I would get sick. In our experience, oils are persistent, even withstanding tooth brushing. He now abstains from eating food containing oils when he knows he will spend time with me. Alternatively, he will wash his face and hands and teeth after eating oils, and then eat an oil free snack with me to avoid cross contamination during kissing.

Pet Food and Other Pet Related Exposure

It may sound ridiculous that pet food could be a danger. However, pet food contains vegetable oils and grease sticks to hands and can be transferred to an eye, mouth or piece of food very easily. I have become sick this way. I wash my hands after handling my cat's food EVERY time, unless I use a tissue to hold the scoop. Another way oil can transfer is through the air when dry food is poured out. I try not to breathe in the particles as I pour.

I do not share dishes with my cat. He has his own special dishes, and I will not to use the same dish washing cloth on my dishes after it had been used on his dish. His dishes are the last to be washed each day; then I throw the dish cloth into the laundry to be cleaned.

My cat likes to lick me. I know dogs do this too. I wash my hands before eating or touching my face.

Cats also bathe and spread oils from their food all over themselves which can then be transferred to wherever they happen to sit. It can be difficult to keep my cat off certain places, like my pillow. I have taken to covering it when I am not using it. I also keep other things that might touch with my face away from him. This includes wash cloths, towels, hats, et cetera. I would really like to find a cat food that does not contain oil but so far that hasn't happened.

Plastic

The truly evil source of oil cross contamination is plastic. Plastic has a chemical structure similar to that of fat, so once it has come in contact with a fat–even the grease from fingers–it will be there forever, despite washing, and will transfer traces to whatever it touches after that. This is unique to fats and oils. Many other substances wash off plastic pretty well. I became ill from using a blender that had come in contact with soy lecithin, even though it had been completely washed.

Wood

Wood can absorb oils. I've had to change out utensils, cutting boards and knife blocks made of wood that have been in contact with vegetable oil.

Whetting Stone

I bought a whetting stone that uses water instead of oil to keep my knives sharp so that I will not accidently transfer oils to my food from sharpening.

About Bread and Other Baked Goods

Before discovering my sensitivity, I ate a lot of bread. I did make bread at home regularly because homemade always tastes better, but I supplemented with store bought.

After I started to be more careful about reading labels, I quickly discovered almost all store-bought bread has some kind of vegetable oil in it. Apparently animal fats are seen as unhealthy in the U.S., so they are almost never used by producers. There was one brand of flat bread I found that did not use oils. I quickly got tired of it.

Once at the local co-op bakery I got very excited when I found a flat bread that did not list any oil on the label. I almost bought it, but first I asked at the counter if they knew any reason that there might be oil in the bread. Thankfully the person who had made it was working and said that she had used canola oil to grease her hands while kneading. I have since learned that it is legal not to list substances that come in contact with food while it is being prepared as long as the substance is under a certain percentage and does not substantially alter the food. Thus, many bakers do not list the grease or cooking spray that is used on the pans.

Before my discovery I ate a lot of cookies and crackers. The soda crackers I could buy all contained vegetable oils. As for other crackers, oil-free offerings at our local stores were very limited. There was one brand of oil-free crackers that I could sort of tolerate. I did try baking crackers, but the results were always disappointing considering the amount of effort involved. I have found some cheese cracker recipes that are okay and are not too difficult.

The cookie offerings were much better. There were half a dozen different brands that used butter instead of vegetable oil. Still, homemade tastes better.

Sadly, all tortillas I have checked use oil either in the dough mixture (flour tortillas) or in the frying process (corn tortillas). I did try making them from scratch. Both corn and flour tortillas are a lot of work to make but they taste marvelous.

It has more recently come to my attention that the bulk yeast that bread is made with contains an oil derivative called sorbitan monostearate. Thus, I would probably not recommend buying any yeast-based breads at this point. At home I always use the yeast that comes in air-tight packets or use wild sourdough to make anything that needs yeast.

Body Products and Environment

When my boyfriend pointed out that the label on his lip balm listed vegetable oil, he sent me down a veritable research rabbit hole.

Because no one else has been talking about oil sensitivity, I basically do a lot of my research about possible reactions and cross contamination on things that have been researched, like gluten sensitivities or peanut allergies, which my sensitivity seems to closely mimic in symptoms.

It turns out that a lot of people with Celiac disease do not get better on a simple gluten free diet. They must remove gluten from everything around them as well. This includes shampoos, nail polish, body lotion, lip gloss, make up, hair spray, soap, detergent, etc. Anything the body comes in contact with, or that touches anything the body comes in contact with, can transmit gluten to the bloodstream.

Ironically, the same products also contain vegetable oils. Laundry products generally leave a residue of oil on clothes, so they will smell 'powder fresh'. Fabric softener sheets feel greasy because they are imbued with oil to carry the scent and calm static. Sunscreens, lotions and most soaps all use vegetable oils to moisturize the skin. When I realized that oils are packaged up by the skin and transported into the bloodstream, I decided to change a lot of my body care products, lotions, laundry care products and household cleaning products. I have not noticed a reaction to vegetable oils used on my skin, but I have experienced oil transfer to my mouth from body products.

I have not been able to find a homemade soap that does not contain some sort of vegetable fat. I did once find a soap that was partly made from lard. All soap is fat that has been saponified, which basically means that the fat has been changed with lye into soap. Eventually, I would like to make my own soap out of lard and tallow, but I have not actually made that happen yet. At this point I buy the highest quality homemade soap I can find and try to stick to ones that use coconut, olive oil, and palm oils.

A few people have written to me and told me that the inhaling oils has been a problem for them. Generally, they mention aerosolized oils from deep fat fryers, but just like flavors, scents are usually carried on oils. (If they don't use oils to carry the scent, they use phthalates, which are nastier). So, although I have not yet had difficulties with smelling French fries, for instance, I do not know how much of my allergic reactions to perfumes is due to the oil carriers. Even essential oils are problematic for me, if they manage to get inside my mouth at all they can and do cause stomach issues.

I have been very cautious of scented dish soaps, Febreze, cleansers, and air fresheners, including air fresheners that plug in, are sprayed, or hang from rear view mirror in cars. I have substituted handmade unscented soap, unscented detergent, vinegar, washing soda, Oxiclean, and baking soda for most of my household needs.

Interestingly, switching away from scented shampoo had the biggest effect on my allergies. My sense of smell returned within a week. Since childhood I had been under the impression that my nose did not work, but it turned out that I had just been congested all the time.

If doing an oil elimination diet, I would recommend reintroducing each of these items separately as they can have a big impact on how people feel.

Flavorings

Flavorings have been a problem for me in general. If you talk to any food scientist–or butcher for that matter–they will tell you that the flavor is in the fat. Thus, most flavorings are made with oils, i.e., fat, including extracts. Even if they do not list an oil (e.g., mint oil) they could have been processed on equipment that has processed oils. One exception to this seems to be natural vanilla (not the fake stuff) which is basically a flower pod/bean soaked in alcohol for an extended period. In effect, the alcohol acts like a solvent and removes the oils from the bean, suspending them and the flavors they contain in liquid. This process uses no heat and is generally kept away from light at well, and because I do not get sick, I have decided that the oils in vanilla are not unsafe for me. Avoiding any listing of 'flavor' on packaging has resolved many stomach issues.

I read a very interesting article online about how manufacturers use flavoring in orange juice ("Freshly Squeezed: The Truth About Orange Juice in Boxes" 2009). The author explained that when orange juice touches oxygen, the volatile flavors vanish, leaving the juice bland and flavorless. Manufacturers add flavor back in. In order to hide this fact, they make the flavorings they add in from the rinds of oranges, so that on the label they can simply list "oranges". Interestingly, in the article, these flavorings were referred to as essential oils, which I know to be a problem for me. At the time I read this article, I was having issues with my stomach that seemed oil related, but I had been unable to find a source of oils. When I stopped drinking orange juice the problems resolved. Later, I found that store bought lemon juice also seems to make me sick. Remember that juice is often added as an ingredient to other foods such as sausages, yogurts, popsicles, and sorbets. These juices might also have the 'flavoring' treatments and could cause problems.

Vitamins and Prescriptions

Vitamins and prescriptions may have been the most insidious place that I found oils. I have taken prescription medications, over the counter medications, and vitamins for years in order to ameliorate the multiple symptoms that I have had to deal with throughout my life. It was very disheartening to find out that many of them have oils or oil derivatives. (See the Hidden Oils section) I discovered that it was not enough to avoid things that say 'oil.' I had to look up each ingredient and find out how it was made and what it was made from to decide if it had oils or not. Oftentimes even things that are not oils per se can be made from oils or are produced as a byproduct of making oils. Think soy lecithin.

As with food, all my vitamins and supplements now contain as few ingredients as possible. It is surprising how many supplements that claim to use "no fillers" contain oils and oil derivatives. For the most part I buy from two herbal companies, Eclectic Institute and Oregon's Wild Harvest. But I have been checking the label for changes each time I buy from them. For the most part I prefer to buy cut and dry herbs in bulk to stuff into capsules myself. The few vitamins I take are mostly bought in bulk and weighed out to be put in capsules or added to my morning probiotic lemonade. I have taken Garden of Life vitamins successfully.

I have found that Aspirin is the only over the counter medication without oil derivatives.

Ironically, allergy medications (which I do not take) contain oil derivatives.

If you take prescription medications it may not be feasible to go off them for a trial elimination diet. Sometimes it can be dangerous, or require a doctor's help in regulating dosages, which can be expensive. Many medications require special withdrawal procedures. Beta blockers, blood pressure medications, antipsychotics, seizure medications, and antidepressants can all be very difficult to wean from. If you are on such medications and the efforts to cease taking them are too daunting, I would recommend simply trying to eliminate as many other sources of oils as possible while continuing to take the required prescription during the diet. I saw a definite improvement in my health with removal of 99% of oils and oil derivatives. Even so, I found that over time my sensitivity to oils increased until even those tiny amounts started to cause problems. Thus, it may be prudent to worry about the oils in prescription medications only after ascertaining that oils are really the problem.

Hints for Cooking Without Oils

People use oils in the kitchen for several different tasks. Many recipes call for oil because it's liquid at room temperature, which most animal fats cannot replicate, and I have found substituting animal fats can throw a wrench into those recipes. Other reasons for using vegetable oils are shelf life, to prevent food from sticking, price, flavor, frying and baking. I have found that as if the recipe does not require the fat to be liquid at room temperature once completed, oil can be exchanged for alternative fats quite easily.

Mayonnaise, pesto, marinades, and salad dressing

Oils stay liquid at room temperature (70 degrees F.). That is why mayonnaise, pesto, marinades, and salad dressing recipes call for oil rather than fat. Still, it is easy enough to make salad dressing with melted solid fats such as butter or lard. They are not as pretty but they taste good. For pesto, it is unnecessary to even melt the fat. I simply chop the ingredients into the fat on a cutting board and it makes a wonderful spread or addition to any soup or sauce. For marinades, I choose to use chicken broth instead of oil. It seems to do a better job of making the meat tender and does not form lumps of cold fat on the meat in the refrigerator. I have not had any luck making mayonnaise with animal fats, but I had no luck making mayonnaise with oil before I found out about my sensitivity, so I have learned to live without it.

Shelf-life

People think that vegetable fats last longer. This is not true. They are usually rancid on the supermarket shelf, but because they have been deodorized no one can tell.

Sticking

Vegetable oils are often used to prevent food from sticking, but I have found fats that are more saturated do a better job. Although butter is high in saturated fats, it also has milk solids that can burn at high temperatures. I have used it successfully to grease bread pans, but I like lard or duck fat better for greasing baking pans and sautéing.

Price

Another reason people cite for preferring oils for cooking is that they are cheaper than animal fats, but that is only the case when comparison shopping. Most meat has animal fat inside at no extra cost, which can be rendered out and saved for future use. So, it can be cheaper to reuse the fats on hand to cook with rather than investing in bottles of oil. Butter is expensive so I tend to mix enough of it in with other fats to flavor foods and help keep the budget low.

Flavor

Some people laud the fact that vegetable oils have a neutral flavor. Vegetable oils are 'neutral' because they are deodorized so no one can tell that they have gone off. Flavor and aroma tell us whether fat is good or spoiled.

Fats are used to add flavor to food. Although fats are not always flavorful themselves, they have the ability to carry flavor within them and disperse it evenly throughout food. This means that anything that has come in contact with fat can flavor it. Connoisseurs generally like flavored fats such as walnut, olive and sesame oils for this reason. Some people do not like meat fats, such as lamb or beef tallow, because the flavor of the animal comes through in the fat. This is up to the individual palette.

Some people honestly do not like the flavor of butter and animal fats. This is mostly because of the way we have been raised. As with most preferences, this is a matter of exposure, as well as hearing ad nauseam that they are "bad for you." We often think that our decision to like or dislike food is immutable, however, that seems to not be the case. I have read that a child must have ten exposures to a food to learn to like it. It has been shown that adults are similar. I personally did not like chicken skin before I discovered my sensitivity. After discovering that chicken skin has lots of good nutrition in it, I found that I could tolerate chicken skin if it was roasted. After that I ate a lot more chicken skin. Now I like the taste of it even if it is cold, and not roasted to crispiness. It is surprising what we can adjust to given time. We think that we eat what we love, but in fact more often we learn to love what we eat.

Frying

People often choose to fry with vegetable oils. Often the term "smoke point" comes up. My reading tells me that cooking food at a high enough temperature to smoke is damaging both to the fats and to the person who consumes them, although the health damage may not show up for decades. If this is the case, fried food is unhealthy and there is no way to make it healthy, although it is probable that frying with vegetable oils or hydrogenated fats is even worse for you than frying with saturated fat. In earlier times, frying was done perhaps once a year—with lard. To avoid damage to fats I cook low and slow. It tastes a little different than fried food, but I find I like it. Sautéing and searing can both be done with animal fats quite easily.

Baking

Cookies, pastries and pie crust recipes often call for hydrogenated fat such as Crisco. Traditionally, recipes for these foods called for a combination of butter (for flavor and stability) and lard (for exquisite tenderness). After trying lard and butter pie crust once (before discovering my oil sensitivity), I swore never return to oil or hydrogenated substitutes, as the taste of lard is far superior.

Chiffon cake recipes call for oil. Here again, I found melted butter worked just fine and tastes marvelous.

Chapter Five: Special Considerations

There are some situations when it comes to avoiding oils that just can't be shoehorned into anywhere else in this book, which is why I put them in their own special chapter. What do you do if you are a vegan? Is an oil elimination diet safe for small children? What do you do if you make a mistake? How do you check with a manufacturer? Is it possible to keep an oil free diet and travel or eat out at restaurants? These are things that I am frequently asked on my blog and I have thought about. I'm sure that there are many more real-life circumstances that people will run into and if your question is not answered here, check my blog. I often post when people ask me new questions. If I haven't addressed your specific problem there feel free to contact me on my blog at https://silverpenblog.wordpress.com I write back when I can.

For Parents Who Suspect Their Child has an Oil Sensitivity

Parents are advised never to do a classic elimination diet for a child because children really need a broad range of nutrition that is not possible on a true (multi item) elimination diet. It is possible to eliminate a *single food* from a child's diet, such as oils, without compromising nutrition levels, as long as the child's diet has enough whole nutritious foods in it.

I will repeat what I said in an earlier chapter: my research has convinced me that, vegetable oils (other than olive oil and coconut oil) are all relatively new to the human diet. None of our great, great grandparents ever ate them. They are not essential for human health, so it is safe not to consume them, as long as we eat a broad diet full of lots of other nutritious foods. By eliminating them from our diet, we are not depriving ourselves of a health food.

If consuming enough Omega 6's and Omega 3's, is a concern, whole foods, including salmon, cod, sardines, eggs, flax seed, and grass-fed beef, provide sufficient Omega 3's and 6's to keep most of us healthy. There are also good fish oil supplements. There is no need to eat vegetable oils to get essential fatty acids.

Oils seem to have a profound effect on my brain. In *The Big Fat Surprise,* Nina Teicholz mentions some interesting studies that show I may not be the only one who's brain is affected by oils. She talks about how some of the toxins in vegetable oils cause cell death. (Teicholz 2014)

Also in a book by Sally Goddard Blythe called *What Babies and Children Really Need* the author talks about how when a dietary ratio of omega 3 to omega 6 fatty acids is not in balance that "trans-fatty acids can become incorporated into brain cell membranes, including the myelin sheath, replacing natural DHA, which then affects the electrical activity of neurons (the power houses of the nervous system)." I take this to mean that trans fats can cause misfiring of the brain in susceptible individuals. (Blythe 2008)

Brain function is essential to a healthy life. It makes it possible to do the things that we want to do. A functioning brain is especially important for growing children. Their brains grow so fast, and they have so much they need to learn, it can be developmentally devastating to have setbacks. There are points during which if the brain does not develop properly there will never be another chance for that development to happen.

Another thing to remember is that children are smaller than adults, so they don't need to eat as much of something to get the same results. Children are often poisoned by amounts that wouldn't have harmed an adult.

I do not say this to scare people, I say this because I have experienced the devastation of having a nonfunctioning brain as a child and I know personally how amazing it was when the oils were removed from my life and I was able to have a fully functioning brain for the first time.

All parents want what is best for their child. If oils are causing problems in a child's brain, a parent should have the opportunity to fix that problem so that their child can be healthy and have a normal life.

Parents have a unique perspective on their child. They can observe the results of oil removal or reduction without their thoughts being clouded by depression or illness, unlike someone in the throes of an oil sensitivity. This means that parents can really see the benefits of partial oil removal. It may be tempting to say "Wow, my kid is doing well enough with partial removal," but I strongly urge parents to remember that if oils are a problem, the oils could be causing more damage than is visible. That damage will have to be repaired, those repairs take time, and they will be hindered by consuming more oils.

Some suggestions for implementing an oil free diet with a child

At the time of this writing my daughter is two and a half. I hate to think of how difficult it would be to change her diet. Currently she eats just like me, oil free and gluten free, and it has been very easy to do since she has never eaten any other way.

Humans tend to eat foods they like because they like them; it's a bit of a viscous cycle really. Eating is a habit, and there are two main schools of thought about how to break habits. One is to go 'cold turkey' and the other is to 'do it gradually'. Either way, researchers have found that forming a new habit is much more lasting than just quitting an old habit. To that end, replacing as many oil laden foods with homemade oil-free versions might make it less stressful and less burdensome for a child. Children are probably like adults in that some kids will be better with change than others, but I think it is safe to say that most would prefer not to change at all without motivation.

Changing diets is always tricky. I remember reading a story about a woman who was concerned about her child not eating vegetables. She told her doctor that no matter what she did her child would not eat anything green. The doctor asked her, "How often to do you eat green vegetables?" The woman tried to think and said, "Not very often, I don't like them that much." Her eyes widened and she said, "Is that why he won't eat them?!"

For me, being around people eating foods I can't eat is isolating, and I am grateful that the people I live with eat like me. It makes sense that children would feel the same way. I've read that often kids that would be unwilling or difficult about changing their lives are often much more open to changes when they help someone else. Parents switching themselves to an oil free diet and asking the child to help them by joining in, might find it easier than saying 'this is for your own good' and continuing to eat oil-laden foods around the child.

It can be difficult to find food outside the home, so I always try to carry a snack when leaving the house. I take food with me wherever I go. Surprisingly once the kitchen is oil free it is not that hard to find something to take. Many of the foods that we think of as lunch foods are easy to pack in a lunch box: sandwiches, nuts, meat, cheese, crackers, chocolate, cookies, veggies, boiled eggs, fruits and even soups. I make bouillon that my mom takes to work for lunch, and it's remarkably portable. In my purse I almost always have a bag of nuts, and if it's going to be a long trip I can throw in some cheese to snack on.

Many blogs discuss how to talk about allergies and food intolerances with children and their caretakers. People often must leave their kids with teachers, babysitters, or even family members. I would recommend reading as many of these resources as possible. I liked The Allergic Child ("AllergicChild," n.d.) but there are many others. The challenges faced by food sensitivity sufferers are remarkably similar even when the foods that they have issues with are completely different.

My mom feels incredibly guilty about the years that I was exposed to the oils, but I do not blame her for not knowing. It can be hard to witness people we love suffering, but suffering is more bearable when we know we are loved. If you do have a child that has an oil sensitivity, keep in mind that accidents happen, and that you are doing your best and that if the oils are your child's particular problem you now have some tools to help them feel better.

Oil Sensitivity and Vegans

Many comments on my oil sensitivity post have been from people who are vegan. From what I understand, vegans do not eat anything that has a face. This includes insects, fish, birds, and reptiles, along with every creature that we traditionally think of as food animals, such as cows, pigs, and deer. This would be hard enough, but vegans also abstain from eating (or using) anything that has come from creatures with a face: such as honey from bees, eggs from chickens, butter from cows and the like. Essentially, they only eat plant products.

I imagine that the reason vegans are seeing problems with eating vegetable oils is because they eat more oil than your average person who eats other types of fats as well, so the effects of a sensitivity to oils would probably show up a lot faster.

I have come up with only one idea for a vegan who finds themselves sensitive to oils to avoid vegetable oils and remain vegan, although there might be other ways.

It is possible not to cook with oils or fats. Foods could be eaten raw or steamed, poached, simmered, or boiled. Using water to cook with has the added benefit of being healthier. Apparently, anything that browns food also adds carcinogens, so by using gentle water-based methods you can avoid that.

To get enough fat, vegans could eat whole fatty plants instead of vegetable oils. There are many fatty plants. Some are well known: avocados, olives, coconut and nuts. But there are some other plants which have some fat that are less well known: cacao nibs, chia seeds, hemp seeds, flax seeds, sunflower seeds, SaviSeeds aka Sacha Inchi, tiger-nut tubers, sedge and purslane.

Eating Out and Travel

For quite some time after I discovered my sensitivity, I continued to go out to restaurants and coffee houses. It is possible to eat out and not consume industrial seed oils. When I traveled to Florida, Las Vegas, and Seattle, I managed to eat at many different places without getting sick. In each case, I researched the menu online beforehand, picked out foods that usually do not contain oils and whenever possible I

68

called ahead, explained my difficulty, and asked about my chosen foods. People were generally sympathetic and helpful. When I arrived at the restaurant I talked to the waiter about my difficulty and had him double check that the food would be prepared without any oil. If I had to ask for a substitution, my food tasted dreadful, but it seemed to work out.

Coffee houses were another matter. It felt like I was playing Russian roulette. Even though I always ordered the same thing. I managed to get sick several times at coffee houses before I realized that the coffeehouse steam wand routinely comes in contact with oil laced soy and rice milks as well as steamed cow's milk. Also, almost all milk used at coffee shops has vitamin D added. So, no matter what I ordered if it was steamed there was always a possibility of cross contamination. I have had iced drinks safely, but I had to remind the staff that they could not stir the cup with any of their implements. I imagine that Americanos and teas would be similar. Eventually, though, I could not bring myself to risk it anymore.

I learned through trial and error that our town was different from big cities. It caters to college kids and penny pinchers, so the restaurant selection is severely limited. Most are fast food joints, offering only prefabricated burgers and sandwiches. No one working there has any idea what is in the food (often they do not have access to the information) and, because the food is prefabricated, it is impossible to accommodate special requests. Doing research online beforehand it is sometimes possible to find one or two foods that do not contain oils. Generally, those items that are high in sugar. Baskin Robbins had two flavors of oil-free ice cream. Orange Julius had some smoothies, and our local self-serve frozen yogurt place had two flavors that I could eat safely. But one cannot live on sugar alone.

It is much harder to find hearty food. I managed to get sick every time I ate out at a restaurant.

My final attempt to dine out in my hometown was for my anniversary. My boyfriend took me to the most expensive restaurant in town. I called ahead. I talked with my waiter. The staff bent over backwards to accommodate me. I got sick. I did wonder about cross contamination, grease in the air, on the pans, and on any surface that could have easily contaminate food cooked in the confines of the kitchen, but I believe that in that instance it may not have been the restaurant's fault. My boyfriend and I did not know about kissing and cross contamination at that point, and the meal he had eaten was not oil free.

By then it was taking longer and longer to recover whenever I slipped up. Three weeks of misery was a lot to pay for a small outing. Eating out was not becoming any easier; quite the opposite, in fact. I was beginning to find it very stressful and so that was the last time I ate out in my hometown.

Although my travel experiences were good, the last time I traveled, I did not eat at restaurants. I drove instead of flying, brought food in a cooler and made sure to stay in a place that had a kitchen. It went well. I have a small child who depends on me and I could not justify the stress of risking my health like that. I'm not sure what I would do if I had to fly.

Calling Manufactures

I do not generally call or e-mail manufacturers about their products, but this can be a way of gathering information. It is good to keep in mind when talking to customer service reps that companies urge their representatives to clam up for fear of legal action if the word allergy is mentioned in a conversation, so it can be helpful not to mention your sensitivity or allergy. It can also be helpful to discuss how things are made and what they are made with. From conversations on blogs and allergy message boards I understand that it can take more than one conversation with a manufacturer to learn everything necessary to be comfortable with a product's safety.

Dealing with Accidental Oil Ingestion

Mistakes seem to be inevitable when it comes to avoiding oils. I have yet to avoid oils for more than eight months at a stretch, even after several years of practice. I always pay for it, too. The stomach symptoms are usually the first thing to heal up, but the mental and emotional symptoms take much longer. I am generally very sick for a week, experience lingering symptoms for three weeks, and only really feel 100% better after two to three months.

I have found a few things that help me avoid some of the more uncomfortable symptoms. If I know I have been exposed, I take 400-500 mg of Alpha Lipoic Acid every hour for the first couple of days. Along with a tablet of vitamin C. It can really limit the symptoms I have to deal with. Eating kefir has been incredibly soothing for my intestinal gas and cramping. I find it can help tremendously with symptoms. I also drink freshly grated ginger tea or take dried ginger pills which helps calm the stomach, reduce gas, nausea and intestinal pain. More recently, I have discovered that a tea made with freshly grated turmeric and ginger with a 1/2 teaspoon of powdered slippery elm added is even more effective than ginger alone. The turmeric helps calm inflammation both in the guts and in the brain, and the slippery elm is wonderful for coating the intestinal lining and preventing further damage. It is not the best tasting tea (understatement). I might try putting the stuff in gel capsules next time to make it more palatable.

I take some extra steps as well. Because the oils damage the intestinal walls, it is important to support that system. If I am experiencing diarrhea, I switch to a modified BRAT diet. BRAT is an acronym for Bananas, Rice, Applesauce, and Toast. I stick to <u>a diet of boiled eggs, homemade bone broth, slices of apple, meat with lots of fat, and vegetables</u> (avoiding the nightshades and legumes). As I get past the acute phase, I add in <u>liver</u>, and more <u>green leafy vegetables</u>, to boost nutrition because nutrition helps the body heal. I also drink <u>nettle tea</u>.

Even if I am not having diarrhea, I stay away from inflammatory and or difficult to digest foods like grains and nuts, and just add in lots of nutritious foods (vegetables, liver, bone broth).

Basically, I figure my body is having an enormous allergy attack, so I take <u>nettles</u>, <u>quercetin</u> and <u>vitamin C</u> every couple of hours because they help with allergies. To calm the inflammation, I take some <u>extra turmeric</u>.

One more supplement has been helping with allergies in general: <u>pancreatin</u>. I started taking it for a completely separate health issue and was surprised by how much weaker my usual allergic reactions to environmental pollutants were. More recently I discovered that pancreatin also helps with the stomach symptoms from oil exposures. It also seemed to help for longer periods of time than the vitamin C or the Alpha Lipoic Acid which is good since vitamin C interferes with its absorption so pancreatin must be taken at least one hour after taking vitamin C or at least two hours before taking more vitamin C.

Every time I have an exposure, the experience is a little different, and I try to keep in mind a few things:

1) I put off making any major life decisions until I feel better. This may seem self-explanatory, but until I realized that I had an oil sensitivity that affects my brain, I made some poor decisions based simply on how awful I was feeling.

2) The symptoms will pass, and I will feel better. Being patient is hard and being sick never seems to get any easier but if I stick to the diet, eventually I recover.

Chapter Six: Avoiding Oils Summary

Eliminating all oils from the diet is the only currently available way to find out conclusively if oils are a problem.

For 100% oil avoidance it is imperative to make all your own food or find someone you trust completely to do it for you.

Oils can be absorbed through the skin and lungs and are found in more than food. They can be found in body products, laundry products, cleaning products, vitamins, herbal supplements, prescriptions, and even in the air we breathe, because of fried foods, added scents, and perfumes. Anything that lists 'fragrance' generally contains oils.

It is important to read labels carefully and avoid ingredients that you do not know or have not researched. Many substances are derived from oils.

Broad terms like 'flavoring' or 'spices' can conceal oils.

Oils are good at cross-contaminating food. They adhere to plastic permanently and contaminate anything that subsequently comes in contact with it. Oils can be smeared on surfaces from other people's hands and can be transferred to your hands and from there to your mouth. Kissing can also transfer oils.

Commercial juices can contain oils.

Oil is on the particles of dry pet food that become airborne and easy to inhale when it is poured out. Pet food, and pets in general, can transfer small amounts of oil. Washing hands and covering surfaces that come in contact with your face or food can reduce exposure from pets and their food.

Conclusion

One of my favorite books features a small child by the name of Jason who was fascinated by the stationary cupboard in the corner of his classroom. His interest may have been because it held all the classroom art supplies, or it might have been because there was a rule that no one but the teacher was allowed to access the stationary cupboard. But Jason tried every way he could think of to get around the rule, including pushing another child in, tripping and falling in, and staying outside and peering in. But the teacher remained firm that he was not allowed in the stationary cupboard.

Having a food sensitivity has been for me much akin that situation. Like Jason, I tried every way I could think of to avoid a completely oil free diet, but eventually I realized I could not eat oils without health consequences.

Fewer of the processed oils bothered me when I was a kid, and they did not bother me as much as they do now. Over the years the sensitivity has increased to the point that a mere trace will cause a severe reaction. This is not untypical of allergy/intolerance reactions: if a person starts out with a bit of an intolerance to chicken eggs, for instance, switching to duck eggs may help for a time, but eventually the duck eggs can start to be a problem.

Even worse, continuing to eat something that your body is mildly intolerant to can train the body to become sensitive or intolerant to other foods. This may be why I have a problem with gluten now.

If a certain type of food causes problems, it seems better to avoid the food entirely, and avoid similar foods to the extent possible. For instance, I *can* have peanut oil–but I do not. I could use it in dressings, mayonnaise, etc., but I have chosen not to, because I see it as only a matter of time before my body starts flagging it as one of the baddies. I do not make a great effort to keep it out of my diet, but it is not in my pantry.

Do I have to stay off oils forever? Will you? In *Food Allergies and Food Intolerance* (Brostoff and Gamlin 2000) the authors suggest that people with food intolerance reintroduce offending foods every six months to determine if the intolerance has cleared up. If no symptoms show, they say that a person can introduce the food back into their diet but never to eat it every day or in large amounts. I personally do not know if I am ever going to feel confident about deliberately exposing myself to see if I have gotten better. My symptoms are too scary.

Others feel the same way. Researchers studying food sensitivities are often stymied when test subjects who have experienced dramatic improvement of their symptoms during the trial removal period suddenly drop out of the study just before the reintroduction of offending food phase of the study.

I haven't flagged animal fats as problem food for three reasons. First, the science I have read about animal fats shows them to be chemically different from oils and very important to body functions. Second, animal fats have been eaten for a long time by humans. My ancestors have been eating animal fat for thousands of years. Lastly, I read a book about harvesting wild plants in which the author said if a food is not helping you, it is hurting you. I feel better when I eat animal fats. I do not feel neutral; I feel better. This, more than anything, is the reason that I choose to eat animal fats.

Ultimately, you are the only person who can decide what foods make you feel better or worse. I hope that this book will help you on your journey.

Short Alphabetized List of Oils and Oil Derivatives

Acetaldehyde

Alpha-linolenic acid

Anhydrous milk fat

Avocado oil

Blue #1

Butter oil

Butter-like spreads

Canola oil, a.k.a. Rapeseed oil

Cis-vaccenic acid

Coconut oil

Docosahexaenoic acid (DHA)

Extra virgin olive oil

Flax oil

Gamma-linolenic acid (GLA)

Gamolenic acid

Glycerol

Glyceryl stearate

Glycerin

Grape seed oil

Hydrogenated oil, or partially hydrogenated

Hypromellose

Hydrogen cyanide

Lauric acid

Light olive oil (always cut with vegetable oils)

Linoleic acid

Magnesium stearate

Margarine

Milk fat

Mono and diglycerides

Nut oils, such as almond, walnut, pecan, and hazelnut

Octadecanoic acid

Oleic acid

Palm oil

Palmitoleic acid

Petroleum jelly

Polyglycerol polyricinoleate PGPR

Polyoxyethylene

Polypropylene glycol stearyl ethers

Polysorbate 20

Polysorbate 80

Safflower oil

Sesame oil

Simethicone

Sodium stearate

Sorbitan monolaurate

Soy lecithin

Soybean oil

Stearic acid

Stearyl alcohols

Sunflower oil

Triglycerides

Vegetable oil

Vegetable glycerin

Vegetable stearin

Bibliography

"AllergicChild." n.d. AllergicChild. https://home.allergicchild.com/.

Blythe, Sally Goddard. 2008. *What Babies and Children Really Need: How Mothers and Fathers Can Nurture Children's Growth for Health and Wellbeing*. Stroud: Hawthorn Press.

Brostoff, Jonathan, and Linda Gamlin. 2000. *Food Allergies and Food Intolerance: The Complete Guide to Their Identification and Treatment*. Inner Traditions / Bear & Co

Overview of research done on allergies and food intolerance before 2000.

Champ, Colin E. 2014. *Misguided Medicine: Second Edition*. Second edition. CDR Health and Nutrition.

Enig, Mary, and Sally Fallon. 2006. *Eat Fat, Lose Fat: The Healthy Alternative to Trans Fats*. Reprint edition. New York: Plume

Sally Fallon is a leader in the Weston Price Foundation's campaign for eating more traditional foods.

Enig, Mary G. 2000. *Know Your Fats□: The Complete Primer for Understanding the Nutrition of Fats, Oils and Cholesterol*. Later Printing Used edition. Silver Spring, MD: Bethesda Pr

Dr. Mary Enig is the expert who testified in Congress in the 70's about the dangers of processed oils. She was ignored.

"Freshly Squeezed: The Truth About Orange Juice in Boxes." 2009. Civil Eats. May 6,

2009. https://civileats.com/2009/05/06/freshly-squeezed-the-truth-about-orange-juice-in-boxes/.

McCullough, Fran, and Dr Barry Sears. 2007. *The Good Fat Cookbook*. 1 edition. New York: Scribner

A lot of information about each fat, good or bad, and how to use good fats in cooking.

Mueller, Tom. 2013. *Extra Virginity: The Sublime and Scandalous World of Olive Oil*. 1 edition. New York: W. W. Norton & Company

An investigation of the olive oil industry. Opened my eyes to the extent of corruption in the food industry and the subsequent danger posed by olive oil contamination.

Nagel, Ramiel, and Timothy Gallagher. 2010. *Cure Tooth Decay: Heal and Prevent Cavities with Nutrition, 2nd Edition*. 2nd edition. Createspace Independent Pub

Talks about the nutrition that whole unprocessed fats offer. A little disorganized but well worth reading.

Niman, Nicolette Hahn. 2014. *Defending Beef: The Case for Sustainable Meat Production*. White River Junction, Vermont: Chelsea Green Publishing

This book has a chapter on why saturated fat is not a health risk and clears up misunderstandings about beef and cows and the damage to the environment that they are responsible for.

Planck, Nina, and Nina Teicholz. 2016. *Real Food: What to Eat and Why*. Reprint edition. Bloomsbury USA

A reassuring and clear explanation of why saturated fats are not bad for you.

Shanahan, Catherine. 2017. *Deep Nutrition: Why Your Genes Need Traditional Food*. 1 edition. New York: Flatiron Books

The book that made me aware that processed fats are not good for anyone. Very thorough scientific explanation of how the various oils and fats act in the body.

"Silver Pen Blog." 2013. Blog. Silver Pen Blog. July 22, 2013. https://silverpenblog.wordpress.com/

This is my personal blog.

Teicholz, Nina. 2014. *The Big Fat Surprise: Why Butter, Meat and Cheese Belong in a Healthy Diet*. 1st Edition edition. New York: Simon & Schuster

A truly in depth look at how saturated fat was demonized, and vegetable oils became a staple of the American diet. Filled with research about both scientific studies and history.

Afterword

Thank you for reading. This Kindle book is meant to be helpful to people who suffer symptoms, physical and mental, after eating or inhaling cooking oils and think that they may have an oil sensitivity. If you would like to ask any questions, please e-mail me at silver_pen@live.com or check out my blog at https://silverpenblog.wordpress.com/.

If you have time, please write a review of this book on Amazon. Good or bad, a review will help others know if the information here might be useful to them.

Made in the USA
Coppell, TX
21 October 2021

64433643R00050